The p̲ ̲ ̲
rocks

Tap into an unlimited and free source of energy

Abdel Levrai

Copyright © 2016 Abdel Levrai

N solutions

All rights reserved.

Disclaimer

The information contained in this book is based upon the research and personal and professional experiences of the author. It is not intended as a substitute for consulting with your physician or other healthcare provider. Any attempt to diagnose and treat an illness should be done under the direction of a healthcare professional.

Although the suggestions in this book are natural, the author is not responsible for any adverse effects or consequences resulting from the use of the ideas or procedures discussed in this book. Should the reader have any questions, the author and publisher strongly suggest consulting a professional healthcare advisor.

INTRODUCTION:

HOW I DISCOVERED THE POWER OF ROCKS

I grew up in a small city in Africa, where there were few people and little to no pollution compared to the big cities all around the world. But life, lead me to travel and live in a big European city, which has nothing to do with my former city in Africa: completely two different worlds.

When I say big city, it means more people, more stress and more pollution and maybe more of other things that I am not aware of. That's why my health took a big hit, and just after few years living in Europe my level of energy dropped dramatically. My level of energy dropped and I was feeling fatigued even when I wasn't doing much.

This left with no choice, but to look for a solution to my problem and thankfully I had the resources to do it. I spent many years reading books, watching videos and attending seminars; all that lead me to test many things to see what really works and what doesn't. I had to change my lifestyle, my diet and so on ...

I always liked natural solutions for the simple reason that they were almost always safer and with no side effect.

To tell you the truth I had some results. My overall health improved as well as my energy level but I wasn't satisfied, I felt that I needed to keep looking for more.

I remember one day I was on the couch watching some reality shows, enable to move or do anything with my days. It was during a period where I was experiencing a low level of energy.

So I thought to myself "why am I feeling tired like that?" and I started to analyze to try to find a reason: it wasn't due to some hard work or activities the days before... maybe it was due to the Wi-Fi and all the electromagnetic field around me.

So I opened my laptop and started doing some research on the impact of electricity and the electromagnetic field on the body. And a book caught my attention, it was: "zapped" by Ann Louise Gittleman.

I ordered the book and then I went on the author's website and I started to read about the solutions that she advocated regarding electronic pollution. And with her I discovered Earthing.

What is Earthing?

Earthing is simply putting your foot, barefoot on the ground and connecting with the earth. The earth contains energy or more exactly negative electrons that benefit your body.

And I told you before, I love natural solutions especially when it involves free energy.

So then I went to the park nearby, took off my shoes and grounded myself and just after two or three minutes I started to feel good, and I started to feel the energy from the earth filling my body. Since that day earthing became my daily routine.

Quickly I felt that it wasn't enough, I wanted to spend more time grounded to the earth, because I became sort of addicted to this good feeling and the energy that earthing provided. It wasn't very convenient because each time I wanted to get grounded, I had to go to the park when my schedule allowed it...

I wanted more energy and more of this good feeling.

Learning about Earthing completely changed my view on nature and earth. Nature can help you get more energy, can heal you and it can make you feel good.

Until one day I was watching an interview of a man who was a sort of life coach who said that he always kept some rocks on his desk to touch. This information caught my attention and I started to ask myself many questions but among them all: is it possible that the rocks contain energy?

1.
THE NEED FOR OTHER SOURCES OF ENERGY

Today we live in a world were energy is depleting, not only external energy like water, oil and so on… but most importantly our inner energy, the energy of our body. Pollution is everywhere and it is increasing. The quality of food is deteriorating with all the chemicals put in it. A modern fast-paced lifestyle, filled with chronic stress, little sleep and lack of physical activity. All that makes us sick and fatigued and leave us with little to no energy to accomplish what we need to do or to enjoy life or the people around us that we love.

That's why people tend to consume many things like coffee, energy drinks and other things that give them a short boost of energy and then leave them empty and more fatigued after their effects are gone.

I think that you get the picture here, there is a clear need for more energy to compensate for what we are losing in our modern world, but also we need to find sources of energy that are natural with no side effects and won't hurt our body afterwards.

The energy business is booming and the demand is increasing. Just look at the many brands of energy drinks that are being sold today. Billions are being made, and those drinks are not very healthy to say the least.

Add to that those sources are not only harmful but they cost money. All that makes them poor sources of energy that need to be avoided.

That's why I think that earthing is amazing because it's free; it's an unlimited source of energy, available everywhere (where there is earth) and natural.

Rocks are exactly the same. A rock is free, is an unlimited source of energy, available everywhere and it is natural.

2.
THE ENERGY OF ROCKS

It is easy to understand where the energy of rocks comes from. Rocks are from the earth and the earth contains energy which means that rocks also contain energy.

By the way if you have never heard of Earthing and you don't understand what I am talking about, I advise you to read the book "Earthing: the most important health discovery ever? "By Clinton Ober. Or better yet, why not go outside and ground yourself and notice how you feel.

I am not a geologist, but from what I learned in high school, I can say that rocks are a little earth glued to form a rock through a process that probably took millions of years. This means that everything that is valid for Earthing is valid for "rocking" ("rocking" like "earthing" got it). All the benefits that you get from the earth you get them from rocks. For example rocks will:

- Defuses the cause of inflammation, and improves or eliminates the symptoms of many inflammation-related disorders.
- Reduces or eliminates chronic pain.
- improves sleep in most cases.
- increases energy.
- Lowers stress and promotes calmness in the body by cooling down the nervous system and stress hormones.
- Normalizes the body's biological rhythms.
- Thins blood and improves blood pressure and flow.
- Relieves muscle tension and headaches.
- Lessens Hormonal and menstrual symptoms.
- Dramatically speeds healing and helps prevent bedsores.
- Reduces or eliminates jet lag.
- Protects the body against potentially Health-disturbing environmental electromagnetic fields (EMFs).

- Accelerates recovery from intense athletic activity.

As it is said in the book "earthing" those are only few benefits and they are probably more.

There is another aspect that I like about it, is that rocks are clean whereas with the earth you need to clean yourself from it especially when it is to dampen. Also rocks can be carried everywhere especially when you travel, and you will still be able to use them and benefit from when you are in a hotel in a big city.

Besides that you won't need too much time to feel energized by rocks. In just three or four minutes you will feel renewed. I know that you don't well understand what I am talking about but I am going to explain everything.

Before there is one more thing that we need to talk about: water!

3.
THE POWER OF WATER

It is said that water is the strongest energy in the world partly because it has the capacity to shape itself in the exact form of the recipient that carries it. For example if you have a cylindrical shaped object filled with water and just near that you have an empty cubical shaped recipient and you pour the water from the first recipient into the second, the water will instantly adapt and take the shape of the second recipient.

Also we all know that water is conductive, it conducts electricity. Let's imagine a bathtub filled with water and you put an electric cable in it then wherever you touch the water you will get electrocuted.

That's not all, water is more sensitive than that. Masaru Emoto, a Japanese researcher who discovered that thoughts and emotions have an effect on water. When he exposes water to a certain thought let's say positive thoughts like thoughts of love, peace or happiness the water would produce a nice crystal when the water was frozen, and when the water was exposed to negative thoughts or intentions then it would yield "ugly" crystals.

This shows us how sensitive and how conductive the water is. This is an important attribute of water that we are going to use to access the energy of rocks.

4.
HOW TO ACCESS THE ENERGY OF ROCKS

We saw how rocks contain energy and where it comes from. We also saw how conductive the water is. Now for us to access the energy of the rocks we simply need to put some rocks in the water. What happens is that the water will instantly conduct the energy of a rock (positive energy) like it conduct electricity. The water will be instantly energized. And this changes everything.

Because the water in your kitchen or your bathroom has lost its energy. It's not a water that comes directly from the river. Usually this water has spent days or maybe weeks in pipelines or stored somewhere and when you use it in your home it's "empty water" with no energy. And you will instantly feel the difference when you use "rocked water" (water with rocks). I will tell you more about it later.

5.
WHAT YOU NEED

All you need is some rocks. Go outside to a forest, a park or to the beach or wherever you think you can find some rocks and pick many rocks of different sizes. Pick rocks of different sizes: the size of fist; others half the size of your fist and one third the size of your fist. Pick around seven rocks. Pick the same type of rocks. For example two or three rocks from a certain type and two to three rocks from another type. When I say type I mean rocks that look alike.

You will also need two containers. The first one will contain the water for you to shower with; for this pick something which has a large opening for you to put the big rocks in it (the size of your fist) and has a cover, to cover the water.

The other container for your drinking water like a jar or something else, also with a top or a cover to keep the water clean.

That's all you need.

6.
HOW TO USE ROCKS

First you clean the rocks that you picked with water and natural soap. Then you put the rocks in the two containers. You should put the big rocks into the container for you to shower with and the smaller ones for the drinking. You can put one rock into each container, that is enough but I prefer to put two rocks or more.

Then you fill them with water:

- For showering:

Once you have filled your container with water, leave it for ten to twenty minutes. The more the better. The best thing to do is to fill it before you go to sleep, that way you let the rocks energize the water all night long.

What you do is you take a regular shower as you do usually, then when you are finished and washed all the soap and the shampoo, you open the container with the "rocked water" and you start washing your body with it. Make sure that the water touches every inch of your body. Pour a little water on any part of your body then rub with your hands.

Start with your arms, pour some water on them and rub them (with your hands) until your shoulders. Then wash your face, your mouth, your neck. Then pour some water on your head (you can take off the rocks) and wash your hair. Pour more water on you and rub your chest, belly, back and genitals. Finally wash your legs and buttocks.

When you are done, don't dry yourself immediately with a towel, let the energized water sink in for a few seconds. Especially when you are not cold. Don't use regular water after that.

Don't leave your container empty when you are finished. Fill it with water and leave for your next shower.

During the winter, when the water is cold you might feel uncomfortable washing yourself with cold water. The solution is to fill your container with half the quantity or two third of the water that you need for you wash with, and before you get under shower and wash yourself as you used to do (with soap, shampoo …) add the second half with hot water, this way you will get cool energized water, that it will be more pleasant to wash yourself with.

Before you wash yourself with the energized water, make sure that you are wet. Pour some "regular" water on you, this way you become more conductive then wash yourself with rocked water as I showed you before.

like to take two showers with the rocked water. One in the morning when I wake up: it gives me energy, focus and alertness during the day. And another one in the evening or before i go to bed: to relax and prepare myself to sleep.

- For drinking:

Put some rocks in the jar, fill it with water and drink from it. It's as simple as that. Even when you buy bottled water, pour the water into the rocked jar. Because almost all the bottled water are empty with no energy in it. After a while you will fill the difference, because the energize water taste differently and has a sort of thickness in it due to its energy, that's regular water doesn't have.

The energized water that you drink will go energize all your internal organs and strengthen them: like your stomach and your kidneys and avoid you many problems that someone might get with this organs.

- In your bath:

When you fill your bathtub with water, add some rocks or one big rock in it. This way all the water will be energized, it will be like taking a bath in a lake or a river. You can do the same in your Jacuzzi.

- In your swimming pool:

You can also place some rocks in your swimming pool; you might need to put bigger rocks in the corners of your pool. This will energize the water and it will be like swimming in a lac or a river because the lac has its water energized by its connection to the earth and rocks. And when you swim in a natural pool like the beach or a river, you will notice the difference: you will be more energized than if you swim in a regular pool. By putting rocks in your pool, you sort of transform your pool into a natural pool (lac, river)...

Other uses:

You can also access the energy of rocks simply by touching it. Hold a rock in your hand, a big one (around the size of your fist), and feel the energy that goes inside your body.

What I like to do is to put a rock on my belly when I am laying down. I find it very energizing. The belly is the center of the body and when you put a rock on your belly you will feel the energy through all your body. This way you can energize yourself while watching TV or talking on the phone or simply resting. Putting a rock on your belly (around the size of your fist) is more powerful than holding it in your hands. It will strengthen your stomach, your abs; help you recover fast and protect you against the electromagnetic field and more.

You can also put a rock somewhere where it hurts of where you have an injury. You can put it on the forehead if you have a headache or toothache; you can also put it on your joints if you fill pain or on a particular muscular muscle

These are the different ways to use rocks and how to access its energy. It is easy implement and the benefits are numerous.

7.
WHEN TO USE THE POWER OF ROCKS

Basically you can use rocked water whenever you want like regular water. But there is few times where it can benefit you the most:

- In the morning

As I said before, showering with rocked water can give you a jump start for the day. It gives you the alertness that you need in order to tackle your daily tasks. It's better than coffee.

- In the afternoon

I like to take a pause in the afternoon for a nap or rest before a work out. And sometimes I don't feel like taking a nap. So I jump under the shower and wash myself with rocked water: I feel refreshed, brand new like I just wake up. It is better than taking a nap, because sometimes when you take a nap you feel lazy or a little bit foggy. The combination of the two (nap + rocked water) is better.

- In the evening:

Showering in the evening helps you to relax and get rid of the fatigue, especially after a work out. It also helps with insomnia: you will sleep earlier and you will sleep better.

- After sex:

Showering with rocked water is excellent after having sex. You will recover from the energy that you lost during sex. This helps you maintain a good level of sexual energy, satisfy your lover while you can still go out there and still have the energy to do what you got to do.

8.
WHAT TO EXPECT FROM USING THE ENERGY OF ROCKS

I remember the first day I showered with rocked water (water with rocks), I felt renewed, energized, alert, focused all day long. What a nice sensation it was. And I still feel the same each day. For me, taking a shower with rocked water is like drinking coffee for many people, it is the thing that's really wake me up: it gives me the jump start or the boost that I need. And it's better than coffee because it has no side effects 100% natural and it takes me only two to three minutes.

What I love the most is the increase of alertness and focus. You feel more present, you feel good and this feeling is priceless. This is because you pour energized water on your head.

Also when I come home after a long day, I jump under the shower and wash myself with rocked water. It makes me feel relaxed and renewed and ready to go again. Thanks to what I taught you, you will be as twice as more productive because you will have more energy. If you think that having a regular shower is relaxing wait until you see how you feel when you shower with rocked water.

It also helps when you are competing or exercising a lot; when you shower with rocked water you recover fast your whole body recovers. Using rocks helps you before exercising and after exercising. It helps recover from injuries, from joints problems ... It also strengthen the body, the muscles, helps you lose weight. I remember that sometimes when I shower I feel my abs strengthened. Rocks

Rocks also help reduce inflammation in your body the same as earthing. They also enhance the mood make you feel good, helps you fight depression.

Drinking rocked water is also important and the benefits are numerous. The water goes inside you and strengthens all your internal organs, specially the kidneys. You know today, many people have kidney problems, and one of the reasons is that the water they drink is empty, with no energy. Bu you, by drinking rocked water you will energize your kidneys every day and help them do their work properly. After a while you will notice the difference between rocked water and regular water, because it tastes different. Rocked water has slightly a different taste and it feels thicker: it is energized.

Many years ago, we used rocked water naturally, by drinking directly from the river and showering in the lac. But today, due to civilization, we have been detached from these natural sources that used to energize our water. By putting rocks in the water, it is a way to go back to how things were before; it is a way to bring nature, the lac, the river into your bathroom or your kitchen.

I can go on and tell you how rocks are good, and all the benefits that you will get from using them, but I think the most important is that you understand what I am talking about, and most importantly is that you go and try what I taught you and you feel all the benefits that I am talking about.

This is a natural, free way to feel good, feel healthy and get more energy. And because it is free that you might underestimate, don't because it might change your life.

CONCLUSION

Discovering this technique of using rocks has really changed my life. It helps me a lot; it helps me deal with the stress, the pollution and the emotional meltdown that you can experience from time to time.

It goes without saying that even when you use the power of rocks, you need to keep on having a healthy lifestyle.

What I like about what I taught you here, is how easy it is to use, the fact that it is free, the fact that I can use it wherever I want and finally the tremendous benefit that I get from it.

I hope that you will give it a try and I hope that what I am giving you in this book will help as much as it does for me or more. And I also hope that you will share it with your beloved ones.

Thank you

Made in the USA
Columbia, SC
08 December 2023